Copyright ©

All rights reserved. No part of this guide may be reproduced in any form without permission in writing from the publisher except in the case of brief quotations embodied in critical articles or reviews.

Legal & Disclaimer

The information contained in this book and its contents is not designed to replace or take the place of any form of medical or professional advice; and is not meant to replace the need for independent medical, financial, legal or other professional advice or services, as may be required. The content and information in this book have been provided for educational and entertainment purposes only.

You agree that by continuing to read this book, where appropriate and/or necessary, you shall consult a professional (including but not limited to your doctor, attorney, or financial advisor or such other advisor as needed) before using any of the suggested remedies, techniques, or information in this book.

TABLE OF CONTENTS

INTRODUCTION

CHAPTER ONE: GOUT BASICS

Cinnamon Baked Apples

Pineapple and Carrot Smoothie

Cherry-Cinnamon Apple Bake

Watermelon-Pineapple Juice

Ginger Potato Soup

Chicken Thyme Casserole

Avocado Cabbage Rolls

Spiced Asparagus

Morning Pie

Cinnamon Roll

Tomato and Avocado Casserole

Cherry Polenta

Enchiladas Frittata

Rosemary Shells

Crockpot Macaroni and Cheese

Marinated Eggplant Dish

Zucchini Casserole

Thyme Stuffed Peppers

Cucumber Boats

Alfredo, Linguine, and Tortellini Casserole

Cornbread Casserole

Ginger Stir Fry and Coconut Rice

Bok Choy Medley

Avocado Tacos

Mex Stackers

Quinoa Chard Pilaf

Nacho Muffins

Mediterranean Zucchini

Spring Rolls

Hummus Zest

Mac and No Cheese

Avocado Fries

Potato Curry

Chicken-Celery Sticks

Quinoa Chard Pilaf

Stuffed Peppers (No Meat)

Veggie and Lentil Bake

Grilled Tomato/Balsamic Veggie Dish

Polenta Arepas (vegan)

Chickpea Casserole

Tempeh Fajitas

Chicken Teriyaki Stir Fry

Kale, Lentil, and Red Onion Pasta

Butter Fettucine

Teriyaki Tofu and Pineapple

Tortillas and Rice

Tofu and Red Bell Peppers

Broccoli Curry

Risotto

Almond and Quinoa Salad

Tofu Fajitas

Vegan Chili

Veggie Burger with Cucumber Salad

Sesame Tofu and Broccoli

Pot Pie Muffin

Stuffed Sweet Potatoes

Veggie Pita

Tofu Kebabs and Cilantro

Chicken Nuggets and Chinese Veggie Salad

Vegan Salad

Pizza (Gout Friendly Version)

Barley and Winter Green Pesto

Garbanzo Cake and Avocado

Veggie Burger Quesadilla

Vegan Paella

Celery Root Soup

Spicy Quinoa and Edamame

Roast Beef Wraps

Black Eyed Peas and Collard Greens and Turnips

Honeyed Corn

Black Bean Quesadilla (Vegan Version)

Baked Tofu and Roasted Pepper

Red Bell Pepper (stuffed)

Baked Pepper Taquitos

White Beans and Chard

Baked Chicken Wings

Miso Soup and Napa Cabbage

Stuffed Pepper Melt

Chinese Porridge (Vegan Version)

Roasted Chicken and White Pepper

Swiss Chard and Garbanzo Beans

Garbanzo Curry

Peaches with Berry Sauce Ice Cream

INTRODUCTION

The diet and lifestyle management tools for gout are not based on any popular diet trend. Instead, the dietary recommendations for gout are deeply rooted in decades of the best available research being conducted worldwide. Remember, adopting healthy lifestyle habits sustainable for the long haul are the key components of an effective gout treatment plan. A well-balanced gout diet can not only lower your risk of an attack, but it can also slow the progression of gout-related joint damage. The key is to choose foods that are low in purine—a chemical compound that, when metabolized, creates the uric acid that triggers gout attacks. Purine is found in many foods, like organ meats, beer, and soda, so these are avoided. Nutritious foods that help your body eliminate uric acid are at the center of an effective diet for managing gout.

A gout diet is generally part of a comprehensive program recommended after you have been diagnosed with the condition. You'll work together with your healthcare provider to manage several lifestyle factors, including diet, weight control, physical activity, and possibly medication to reduce the frequency and intensity of gout attacks.

The recipes contained in this book are not intended to be any type of Medical advice. ALL individuals must consult their Doctors first and should always receive their meal plans from a qualified practitioner. These recipes are not intended to heal, or cure anyone from any kind of illness, or disease.

CHAPTER ONE: GOUT BASICS

What is Gout

Gout is a form of arthritis that affects over three million Americans each year. Also known as gouty arthritis, the disease is caused by the formation of uric acid crystals in a joint (most often the big toe), triggering severe pain, redness, and tenderness. While certain factors, like genetics or kidney disorders, may predispose you to gout, diet, alcohol, and obesity can also contribute. For some people gout looks like a sudden swelling at the base of the big toe. The big toe is the most common place for a gout attack to happen, though gout can attack many different joints in the body.

People with gout typically experience flare-ups, or attacks, of symptoms followed by periods with no symptoms. These attacks typically last 3 to 10 days.

Some people go months or even years without a gout attack after having one. In other people, attacks may become more frequent over time.

Gout can be difficult to diagnose. Once it's diagnosed, it can be treated with medication and lifestyle changes.

Treatment can include over-the-counter (OTC) and prescription drugs to alleviate pain and reduce uric acid levels. You can further minimize the frequency of attacks by losing weight, exercising regularly, and avoiding trigger foods.

Gout Symptoms

The symptoms of gout tend to be progressive and will worsen over time if left untreated. The severity and recurrence of symptoms are largely related to the stage of the disease.

Asymptomatic gout is the period prior to your first attack. It is during this time that the persistent elevation of uric acid in your blood will cause urate to form crystals. While you will not experience any symptoms at this stage, the gradual accumulation of crystals will almost inevitably lead to an attack.

Acute intermittent gout is the stage when you will start to experience attacks lasting anywhere from three to 10 days. The attacks (most commonly affecting the big toe but also the knee, ankle, heel, midfoot, elbow, wrist, and fingers) will cause sudden and extreme pain accompanied by swelling, stiffness, redness, fatigue, and occasionally mild fever.

Chronic tophaceous gout is an advanced stage of disease in which the urate crystals consolidate into hardened lumps called tophi. The formation of these mineralized masses can progressively erode bone and cartilage tissue and lead to chronic arthritis and joint deformity.

Complications of untreated gout include kidney stones and the deterioration of kidney function.

Causes of Gout

Gout is caused by too much uric acid in the bloodstream and accumulation of urate crystals in tissues of the body. Uric acid crystal deposits in the joint cause inflammation of the joint leading to pain, redness, heat, and swelling. Uric acid is normally found in the body as a byproduct of the way the body breaks down certain proteins called purines. Causes of an elevated blood uric acid level (hyperuricemia) include genetics, obesity, certain medications such as diuretics (water pills), and chronic decreased kidney function (kidney disease).

While certain factors can predispose you to the disease, such as genetics or chronic kidney disease, others like diet, alcohol, and obesity can contribute just as profoundly.

While men are more likely to have gout than women, the risk in women can significantly increase after menopause.

Dietary Causes

Unlike other forms of arthritis, gout is caused by abnormalities in body metabolism rather than the immune system. The risk of gout is related to multiple factors—genetic, medical, and lifestyle—that together contribute to a rise in uric acid levels in the blood, a condition we refer to as hyperuricemia.

The foods we eat can play a significant role in the development of gout symptoms. This is due in large part to an organic compound found in many foods called purine. When consumed, purine is broken down by the body and converted into the waste product, uric acid. Under normal circumstances, it would be filtered out of the blood by the kidneys and expelled from the body through urine.

If uric acid is formed faster than it can be excreted from the body, it will begin to accumulate, eventually forming the crystals that cause attacks. Certain foods and beverages are common triggers for this. Among them:

• High-purine foods are considered a major risk factor for gout. These include foods like organ meats, bacon, veal, and certain types of seafood.

• Beer is especially problematic as it is made with brewer's yeast, an ingredient with an extremely high purine content. But any form of alcohol, in general, can increase risk of gout attack.

• High-fructose beverages, including sodas and sweetened fruit drinks, can cause hyperuricemia as the concentrated sugars impair the excretion of uric acid from the kidneys.

Genetic Causes

Genetics can play a significant role in your risk of gout. Hereditary hyperuricemia is one such example, caused by SLC2A9 and SLC22A12 mutations that lead to the impaired renal (kidney) excretion of uric acid.

The inability to maintain equilibrium between how much uric acid is produced and how much is expelled will ultimately lead to hyperuricemia.

Other genetic disorders linked to gout include:

- Hereditary fructose intolerance
- Kelley-Seegmiller syndrome
- Lesh-Nyhan syndrome
- Medullary cystic kidney disease

Medical Causes

There are certain medical conditions that can predispose you to gout. Some directly or indirectly affect renal function, while others are characterized by an abnormal inflammatory response, which some scientists believe may promote uric acid production.

Some of the more common medical risk factors include:

- Chronic kidney disease
- Congestive heart failure
- Diabetes
- Hemolytic anemia

- Hypertension (high blood pressure)
- Hypothyroidism (low thyroid function)
- Lymphoma
- Psoriasis
- Psoriatic arthritis

Other medical events are known to trigger a gout attack, including a traumatic joint injury, an infection, a recent surgery, and a crash diet (possibly through rapid changes in blood uric acid levels).

As with any disease or medical conditions, it's important that those with gout adopt lifestyle choices that minimize the intensity of pain that they feel from their condition. One of those lifestyle changes has to be a change in diet, because there are certain foods that can make gout worse but also others that can make it better.

PART TWO: RECIPES

The worst foods for gout are those that are rich in purine, such as red meats, seafood, or breads, because purine is made up of uric acids that if released into the body will only increase the swelling around the joints and thus make the pain worse.

On the flip side of things, anti-purine foods will allow you to enjoy a delicious meal while avoiding the ingredients that can cause your pain to flare up. If you've been suffering from gout for too long and need to find meals that you can enjoy while simultaneously minimizing your pain, then you've come to the right place.

Curried Carrot, Potato, and Ginger Soup

Serves: 5

Preparation Time: 30 Minutes

Ingredients

• 2 Teaspoons of Canola Oil

• 1 Tablespoon of Sugar

- ½ Cup of Shallots
- 3 Cups of Sweet Potato (peeled)
- 1 Tablespoon of Ginger
- 2 Teaspoons of Curry Powder
- 3 Cups of Chicken Broth
- Salt and Pepper

Directions

1. Begin by heating the oil in a pan over a medium flame
2. Place shallots into the pan and sauté for three minutes
3. Add carrots, ginger, potato, and curry and mix together; cook this mixture for 2 minutes
4. Pour in broth and bring it to a bowl
5. Place a lid over the bowl, lower the heat, and allow the mixture to simmer for twenty minutes
6. Add salt and pepper to taste
7. Pour the resulting soup into a bowl and allow it to cool before serving

Nutritional Information

- Calories: 144

- Fat: 2.3g
- Carbs: 27.3g

Waldorf Salad

Serves: 4

Preparation Time: 10 Minutes

Ingredients

- 2 Tablespoons of Mayonnaise
- 1 Tablespoon of Lemon Juice
- 8 Leaves of Lettuce
- ¼ Cup of Celery
- ¼ Cup of Walnuts
- 1 Cup of Grapes
- 2 Apples
- 1/3 Cup of Cranberries (dried)

Directions

1. Mix the lemon juice, mayonnaise, grapes, apples, and cranberries together in a bowl

2. Add celery and walnuts and mix thoroughly again

3. Pour mixture over lettuce leaves

4. Either serve immediately or refrigerate for up to two hours

Nutritional Information

- Calories: 153
- Fat: 6g
- Carbs: 26g
- Sodium: 72mg
- Calcium: 28mg

Amaranth Porridge

Serves: 2

Preparation Time: 40 Minutes

Ingredients

- 2/3 cups of Amaranth Grain
- 2 Cups of Water
- 1 Tablespoon of Honey
- ¼ Hemp of Pumpkin Seeds
- ½ Cup of Blueberries
- 1 Pear (chopped)

Directions

1. Mix the amaranth and water together in a skillet

2. Place the skillet over a medium to high flame and allow it to boil before bringing it back to a low flame

3. Allow the mixture to simmer for twenty five minutes and stir periodically

4. Remove the mixture from the flame and add the rest of the ingredients except for the pear and blueberries

5. Pour the resulting porridge into bowls and add the blueberries and pear

6. Serve

Nutritional Information

- Calories: 460
- Carbs: 63g
- Sugar: 22g
- Fat: 12 g

Kale Chips

Serves: 8

Preparation Time: 2 Hours and 30 Minutes

Ingredients

- 2 Bunches of Washed Kale

- 1 Cup of Sweet Potato (grated)

- 1 Tablespoon of Honey

- 2 Tablespoon of Yeast

- 1 Lemon

- 1 Cup of Cashews

- 2 Tablespoon of Water

- Salt and Pepper

Directions

1. Set your oven to one hundred and fifty degrees Fahrenheit

2. Set the kale into a bowl

3. Mix the rest of the ingredients together in a blender and process it until it has become smooth

4. Pour the processed ingredients over the kale and mix together

5. Place what you have prepared so far on parchment paper and set it in the oven

6. Keep the mixture in the oven for two hours

7. Remove from oven and store in a container until serving

Nutritional Information

- Calories: 190
- Carbs: 26g
- Fiber: 5g
- Sugar: 4g
- Fat: 8g

Beet Salad

Serves: 4

Preparation Time: 15 Minutes

Ingredients

- 1 Beet (grated)
- 1 Carrot (grated)
- 1 Apple
- 2 Tablespoons of Lemon Juice
- 2 Tablespoons of Pumpkin Seed Oil

- 1 Tablespoon of Almonds
- 4 Cups of Lettuce

Directions

1. Mix all of the ingredients, except for the lettuce, in a bowl

2. Place one cup of lettuce over every plate, for four plates total

3. Pour the mixed ingredients over the lettuce plates and serve

Nutritional Value

- Calories: 130
- Carbs: 12g
- Fat: 9g

Kiwi Kale Smoothie

Serves: 1

Preparation Time: 10-15 Minutes

Ingredients

- 2 Kiwifruits
- 2 Cups of Kale
- 5 Ounces of Water

- 1 Mango

- 1 Orange

Directions

1. Put all of the ingredients together in a blender and process until it has mix together into a smoothie

2. Pour into a glass and serve

Nutritional Value

- Calories: 354

- Protein: 8g

- Carbs: 86g

Raw Pad Thai

Serves: 4

Preparation Time: 20 Minutes

Ingredients

- 1 Zucchini

- 1 Green Onion

- 1 Carrot

- ½ Cup of Bean Sprouts

- ½ Cup of Cauliflower Florets

- ½ Cup of Cabbage
- 2 Tablespoons of Tahini (for sauce)
- 2 Tablespoons of Almond Butter (for sauce)
- 1 Tablespoon of Honey (for sauce)
- 1 Tablespoon of Tamari (for sauce)
- 1 Tablespoon of Lemon Juice (for sauce)
- ½ Teaspoon of Ginger Root (for sauce)
- ½ Teaspoon of Garlic (for sauce)

Direction

1. Run the zucchini and the carrots through a vegetable peeler to make noodles

2. Place the noodles into a bowl and top them off with the rest of the vegetables

3. Take all of the sauce ingredients and mix together in a bowl; whisk until thick

4. Pour the completed sauce over the vegetables and mix them

thoroughly together; the sauce should thin out

5. Pour into bowls and serve

Nutritional Value

- Calories: 140

- Carbs: 14g

- Sugar: 8g

- Fat: 9g

- Sodium: 510mg

Key Lime Pie

Serves: 8

Preparation Time: 45 Minutes

Ingredients

- 1 Cup of Shredded Coconut (for crust)

- 1 Cup of Walnuts (for crust)

- ½ Cup of Pitted Dates (for crust)

- 1/4 Teaspoon of Salt (for crust)

- 3 Avocados (for filling)

- ½ Cup of Honey (for filling)

- 1 Teaspoon of Lime Juice (for filling)

- 3 Tablespoon of Lime Juice (for filling)

- Kiwi Slices as Desired

Directions

1. Mix the walnuts, coconuts, and salt together and process until grounded

2. Add dates and process again

3. Press the mixture into the sides of a pie plate with the aid of a spoon to make the crust

4. Freeze the crust for 15 minutes

5. Place all of the ingredients for the filling in a processer and process until they have smoothed

6. Pour the filling into the crust, and add kiwi slices as desired

7. Place in the refrigerator for twenty minutes

8. Serve

Nutritional Value

- Calories: 390
- Carbs: 37g
- Fiber: 8g
- Sugars: 26g
- Fat: 28g
- Sodium: 70mg

Melon Mango Smoothie

Serves: 1

Preparation Time: 15 Minutes

Ingredients

- 2 Cups of Cantaloupe

- 2 Leaves of Chard

- 6 Strawberries

- 2 Mangoes

- 5 Ounces of Water

- 1 Stalk of Celery

- 2 Cups of Spinach

Directions

1. Pour the water into a blender and add each of the ingredients

2. Process until it has mixed well into a liquid smoothie form

3. Pour into a glass and serve

Nutritional Value

- Calories: 384

- Protein: 8g

- Fat: 2g

Kale Salad

Serves: 4

Preparation Time: 20 Minutes

Ingredients

- 6 Cups of Kale

- ½ Lemon

- 1 Pinch of Basil

- 1 Pinch of Salt

- 1 Tablespoon of Olive Oil

- 1 Cucumber

- 2 Tablespoons of Green Onion

- 2 Tablespoons of Red Onion

- 1 Clove of Garlic

- ¼ Cup of Olives

Directions

1. Cut the kale into thin strips

2. Steam the kale strips for 6 minutes

3. Transfer the steamed kale strips to a bowl

4. Mix olive oil, salt, basil, and lemon with the kale thoroughly together

5. Add the rest of the ingredients and mix again

6. Serve

Nutritional Value

- Calories: 150

- Carbs: 13g

- Fat: 10g

- Sugar 1g

Pineapple-Grapefruit Smoothie

Serves: 1

Preparation Time: 15 Minutes

Ingredients

- 1 Banana (peeled)

- 5 Ounces of Water

- ½ Cup of Cilantro

- ½ Cucumber

- 1 Cup of Pineapple

- ½ Grapefruit

Directions

1. Place all of the ingredients into a blender and process until in smoothie form

2. Pour into a glass and serve

Nutritional Value

- Calories: 262

- Proteins: 46g

- Carbs: 67g

Cinnamon Baked Apples

Serves: 4

Ingredients

- ½ Cup of Nuts

- ¼ Cup of Cranberries

- 4 Apples

- ¼ Teaspoon of Cloves

- ½ Teaspoon of Nutmeg

- 1 Teaspoon of Cinnamon

- 1 Teaspoon of Ginger Root

- 2 Dates

- 1 Cup of Apple Juice

- ¼ Cup of Honey

Directions

1. Preheat your oven to 325 degrees Fahrenheit

2. Mix the cranberries, nuts, ginger root, dates, and spices together in a bowl

3. Cut out the core from each apple, and then fill up the resulting hole with the mixture

4. Cover the apples in honey and place on a baking dish

5. Pour apple juice around and over the apples

6. Bake for a half hour

7. Remove from oven and serve

Nutritional Value

- Calories: 350

- Carbs: 69g

- Sugar: 56g

- Fat: 10g

Pineapple and Carrot Smoothie

Serves: 1

Preparation Time: 15 Minutes

Ingredients

- 1 Orange

- 2 Cups of Pineapple

- 2 Carrots
- 2 Tablespoons of Chia Seeds
- 8 Ounces of Water
- 2 Cups of Spinach
- ½ Teaspoon of Ginger

Directions

1. Place all of the ingredients in a blender and process until it has liquefied thoroughly into smoothie form

2. Pour into a glass and serve

Nutritional Value

- Calories: 337
- Protein: 8g
- Carbs: 52g

Cherry-Cinnamon Apple Bake

Serves: 2

Ingredients

- 1 Cup of Cherries
- 2 Apples
- 1 Tablespoon of Cinnamon

- ½ Teaspoon of Nutmeg

- 3 Tablespoons of Raisins

Directions

1. Preheat your oven to 375 degrees Fahrenheit

2. Mix all of the ingredients thoroughly together

3. Set the mixture on an oven baking dish and bake for 45 minutes

4. Remove from oven and serve

Nutritional Value

- Calories: 190

- Fat: 0.5g

- Sugar: 38g

Watermelon-Pineapple Juice

Serves: 1

Ingredients

- 1/3 Pineapple

- 2 Slices of Watermelon

- 1 Inch of Ginger Root

Directions

1. Cut the core out of the pineapple

2. Place all of the ingredients into a juicer and process until in liquefied form

3. Pour into ice glasses and serve

Nutritional Value

- Calories: 300
- Protein: 21g

Ginger Potato Soup

Serves: 2

Preparation Time: 40 Minutes

Ingredients:

- 1 Tablespoon of Olive Oil
- 2 Sweet Potatoes
- 1 Clove of Garlic
- 2 Teaspoon of Ginger
- 4 Leaves of Mint
- 1/3 Teaspoon of Turmeric
- 2 Cups of Vegetable Broth

Directions

1. Pour the olive oil into a food processor

2. Peel the sweet potatoes and place them into the processor next

3. Add garlic gloves, turmeric, mint leaves and ginger next

4. Process the mixture together

5. Pour into a pot and set it over a medium flame for 30 Minutes

6. Serve

Nutritional Value

• Calories: 140

• Fat: 4g

• Carbs: 27g

• Protein: 4g

Chicken Thyme Casserole

Serves: 2

Preparation Time: 50 Minutes

Ingredients

• 1 Cup of Dark Chicken Meat

• 2 Cups of Brown Rice

• ½ Cup of Water

- ½ Cup of Peas
- ½ Cup of Carrots
- 2 Teaspoons of Thyme
- 1 Teaspoon of Celery
- Salt and Pepper

Directions:

1. Brown the pieces of chicken in an oven

2. Mix brown rice, water, carrots, salt and pepper, celery, thyme, and peas together with the chicken in a pot

3. Set the bowl over a high flame until it boils

4. Reduce the flame to low and allow the mixture to simmer for 30 Minutes

5. Serve

Nutritional Value

- Calories: 143
- Carbs: 34.6mg
- Protein: 16.5g
- Fat: 46.4g

Avocado Cabbage Rolls

Serves: 1

Preparation Time: 25 Minutes

Ingredients

- 1 Tablespoon of Olive Oil

- 1 Avocado

- 1 Tablespoon of Apple Cider Vinegar

- 1 Head of Cabbage

- ½ Tablespoon of Chili Powder

- 1 Small Onion

Directions

1. Preheat your oven to 425 degrees Fahrenheit

2. Add 1 tablespoon of olive oil to a skillet

3. Saute onion in the olive oil for a minute

4. Add chili powder, apple cider, vinegar, and avocado and mix

5. Fill up each cabbage leaf with the mix

6. Set on baking tray and bake for 12 minutes

7. Serve

Nutritional Value

- Calories: 75

- Fat: 3.5g
- Protein: 4.6g
- Carbs: 31mg

Spiced Asparagus

Serves: 3

Preparation Time: 35 Minutes

Ingredients

- 12 Asparagus
- 1 Tablespoon of Olive Oil
- 1 Cup of bread Crumbs
- 1 Cup of Parmesan
- ½ Tablespoon of Jalapeno Powder

Directions

1. Preheat your oven to 400 degrees Fahrenheit

2. Mix olive oil, bread crumbs, jalapenos, and parmesan together in a bowl

3. Place asparagus into the mixture until cover

4. Set on a baking tray and bake for 20 minutes

5. Serve

Nutritional Value

- Calories: 89
- Fat: 3.4g

Morning Pie

Serves: 2

Preparation Time: 2 Hours and 30 Minutes

Ingredients

- 1 Tablespoon of Olive Oil
- 1 Teaspoon of Garlic
- 1/3 Cup of Salsa
- 1 Roll of Biscuit Dough
- ½ Cup of Cheddar cheese
- 4 Egg Whites

Directions

1. Mix garlic, salsa, and egg whites thoroughly together

2. Cover with pieces of your biscuit dough

3. Top off with cheese

4. Cook in a crock pot at medium heat for two hours

5. Cool and serve

Nutritional Value

- Calories: 321

- Fat: 34g

Cinnamon Roll

Serves: 2

Preparation Time: 2 Hours

Ingredients

- 1 Cinnamon Roll

- 2 Tablespoons of Melted Butter

- 2 Cups of White Sugar

- ¾ Tablespoon of Brown Sugar

- 23/ Cup of Lemon Juice

- 4 Teaspoons of Cinnamon

- 1 Cup of Pecan Pieces

Directions

1. Mix the white sugar and lemon juice together in a bowl

2. In a second bowl, mix the brown sugar, pecan, and cinnamon

3. Roll the cinnamon dough into a flat sheet piece and pour melted butter over it

4. Cook for one hour in a crock pot on high

5. Remove from crock pot and coat with both sugar mixtures

6. Cook on high for another half hour

7. Serve

Nutritional Value

- Calories: 456

- Fat: 46g

- Carbs: 46mg

- Protein: 16g

Tomato and Avocado Casserole

Serves: 2

Preparation Time: 30 Minutes

Ingredients

- Cubed Ciabatta Bread

- 1 Tablespoon of Olive Oil

- 1/3 Cup of Scallions

- 1 Avocado

- ½ Cup of Tomatoes
- 3 Leaves of Basil
- 1 Cup of Mozzarella

Directions

1. Preheat your oven to 350 degrees Fahrenheit

2. Mix together olive oil, tomatoes, scallions, basils, and avocado in a bowl

3. Place the Ciabatta bread in a dish and top with the above mixture and cheese

4. Bake for 20 minutes

5. Serve

Nutritional Value

- Calories: 87
- Fat: 14g
- Carbs: 9g
- Protein: 11g

Cherry Polenta

Serves: 3

Preparation Time: 1 Hour

Ingredients

- 1 Tablespoon of Butter
- Olive Oil as Desired
- 2 Cups of Polenta
- 2 Cups of Milk
- 1 ½ Cup of Cherries

Directions

1. Mix polenta, butter, olive oil, and milk together and stir

2. Bring this mixture to a boil over a high flame

3. Reduce the heat and allow it to simmer for 40 minutes

4. Add cherries and serve

Nutritional Value

- Calories: 136
- Fat: 45g
- Carbs: 31mg
- Proteins: 7g

Enchiladas Frittata

Serves: 3

Preparation Time: 30 Minutes

Ingredients

- 6 Egg Whites
- Olive Oil as Desired
- ½ Can of Sodium
- 1/3 Cup of Salsa
- 1 Teaspoon of Hot Sauce
- 2/3 Tablespoon of Chili Powder
- 1 Teaspoon of Cumin
- 1 Teaspoon of Celery
- 1 Package of Cheddar cheese

Directions

1. Prepare a skillet over a medium heat and melt butter with olive oil

2. Mix tomatoes, egg whites, salsa, hot sauce, cumin, chili powder, and celery

3. Top with cheese and cook over skillet for 20 minutes before serving

- Calories: 101
- Fat: 10mg
- Carbs: 34mg
- Protein: 9g

Rosemary Shells

Serves: 2

Preparation Time: 40 Minutes

Ingredients

- 1 Tablespoon of Olive Oil
- 1 Package of Stuffed Shells
- ½ Cup of Ricotta Cheese
- 1 Tablespoon of Rosemary
- ½ Cup of Tomatoes

Directions

1. Preheat oven to 400 degrees Fahrenheit

2. Pour in olive oil into a dish

3. Place the shells on dish with their open sides up

4. Mix cheese, tomatoes, and rosemary and pour the mixture into the open shells

5. Cook for 30 minutes before serving

Nutritional Value

- Calories: 78
- Fat: 32g

Crockpot Macaroni and Cheese

Serves: 3

Preparation Time: 2 Hours

Ingredients

- 1 Tablespoon of Olive Oil
- 1 Tablespoon of Butter
- 1 Teaspoon of Garlic
- 1 Tablespoon of Sriracha Sauce
- 1 Teaspoon of Onion Powder
- 1 Cup of Chicken Bouillon
- ½ Cup of Milk
- 8 Ounces of Macaroni
- 1 Cup of Monterey Jack Cheese
- ½ Cups of Bread Crumbs

Directions

1. Mix all of the ingredients except for the macaroni and cheese in a crock pot

2. Add the macaroni and cheese and stir thoroughly together

3. Cook over a low heat for an hour and a half before serving

Nutritional Value

• Calories: 178

• Fat: 59g

• Carbs: 56mg

Marinated Eggplant Dish

Serves: 3

Preparation Time: 4 Hours and 30 Minutes

Ingredients

• 1 Tablespoon of Olive Oil

• ½ Tablespoon of Butter

• 1 Teaspoon of Worcester Sauce

• 1/3 Cup of Honey

• 1/3 Cup of Brown Sugar

- 1 Teaspoon of Black Pepper
- 1 Tablespoon of Ginger Powder
- 1 Onion
- 1 Cup of Eggplant

Directions

1. Mix olive oil, honey, sugar, ginger, pepper, and butter in a bag to form a marinade

2. Place the onion and eggplant in the marinade and set it in a refrigerator for four hours

3. Remove from refrigerator and simmer over a high flame for 5 minutes before serving

Nutritional Value

- Calories: 111
- Fat: 15g

Avocado Medley

Serves: 2

Preparation Time: 35 Minutes

Ingredients

- ¾ Tablespoon of Olive Oil
- 1 Cup of Brown Rice

- ¾ Cup of Water
- Garlic to taste
- 1 Tomato
- 1 Onion
- 1 Cup of Egg Plant
- 1 Avocado
- ¼ Cup of lemon Juice
- 1 Tablespoon of Basil

Directions

1. Pour the olive oil in a pot and warm over a high flame

2. Saute tomato, eggplants, avocado, and onion in olive oil for 2 minutes

3. Pour lemon juice, water, rice, and garlic into the mixture and boil while stirring

4. Reduce heat and allow it to simmer for 25 minutes before serving

Nutritional Value

- Calories: 57
- Fat: 16g
- Carbs: 25mg

* Protein: 5g

Zucchini Casserole

Serves: 3

Preparation Time: 25 Minutes

Ingredients

* 3 Zucchinis

* 1 Cup of Mozzarella

* 1/3 Cup of Olive Oil

* ½ Tablespoon of Parsley

* 1 Tablespoon of Rosemary

Directions

1. Preheat oven to 400 degrees Fahrenheit

2. Place Zucchini in a bowl, and mix it with the rest of the ingredients

3. Bake for 20 minutes before serving

Nutritional Value

* Calories: 77

* Fat: 43g

* Carbs: 39mg

* Protein: 6.5g

Thyme Stuffed Peppers

Serves: 2

Preparation Time: 3 Hours

Ingredients

- 2 Bell Peppers
- 1 Tablespoon of Olive Oil
- ½ Cup of Rice
- 1 Can of Tomatoes
- 1 Cup of Beef Brother
- ½ Tablespoon of Thyme
- ½ Cup of Parmesan

Directions

1. Remove seeds from peppers and place peppers inside a crock pot

2. Mix rice, broth, tomatoes, and thyme together

3. Place the mixture into the open peppers and sprinkle with cheese

4. Cook over a low heat for three hours before serving

Nutritional Value

- Calories: 134

- Fat: 24g

- Carbs: 21mg

Cucumber Boats

Serves: 2

Preparation Time: 20 Minutes

Ingredients

- 2 Cucumbers

- 1 Tomato

- 1 Shallot

- 1 Tablespoon of Italian Dressing

- ½ Tablespoon of Chia Seeds

Directions

1. Preheat oven to 325 Degrees Fahrenheit

2. Cut the cucumbers in half and lay with the open side up

3. Mix tomatoes, shallot, dressing, and cheese together and place on the open cucumbers; top with seeds

4. Bake for 15 Minutes before serving

- Calories: 87
- Fat: 9.4g

Alfredo, Linguine, and Tortellini Casserole

Serves: 1

Ingredients

- 1 Tablespoon of Olive Oil
- 1 Teaspoon of Garlic
- ½ Shallot
- 2 Cups of Cheese Tortellini
- 1 Cup of Alfredo Sauce
- 1 Teaspoon of oregano
- 1 Cup of Italian Cheese
- 8 Ounces of Linguine

Directions

1. Preheat Oven to 350 degrees Fahrenheit

2. Cook Linguine according to instructions on the package

3. Mix Alfredo sauce, tortellini, oregano, and Italian cheese together

4. Pour into a dish and bake for 30 minutes

Nutritional Value

- Calories: 213
- Fat: 25g

Cornbread Casserole

Serves: 3

Preparation Time: 40 Minutes

Ingredients

- 2 Cups of Green Beans
- ½ Cup of Corn
- ½ Cup of Carrots
- 3 Cups of Cornbread (crumbled)
- 1 Teaspoon of Sage
- ½ Teaspoon of Cloves

Directions

1. Preheat oven to 350 degrees Fahrenheit

2. Mix butter, beans, corn, carrots, cloves, and sage in a bowl

3. Place crumbled cornbread on the bottom of a dish

4. Place mixture over the cornbread

5. Cook for 30 Minutes

Nutritional Value

- Calories: 345

- Carbs: 56g

- Fat: 47g

- Protein: 24g

Ginger Stir Fry and Coconut Rice

Serves: 1

Ingredients:

- ½ Teaspoon of Corn Starch

- ½ Cloves of Garlic

- ½ Teaspoon of Ginger Root

- 2 Teaspoons of Olive Oil

- 1 Tablespoons of Red Bell Pepper

- 2 Tablespoons of Carrots

- 1 Teaspoon of Soy Sauce

- Water

- ½ Tablespoon of Chopped Onion

- ¼ Cup of Jasmine Rice

- ¼ Cup of Coconut Milk

- ¼ Cup of Hot Sauce

Directions

1. Place rice, coconut milk, and water in a pot and boil over a high flame

2. Reduce to low heat and allow the mixture to simmer for 15 minutes

3. Mix corn starch, ginger, garlic, and olive oil together

4. Add peas, broccoli, carrots, and bell pepper together

5. Heat olive oil over a medium heat and sauté vegetables for 1 minute

6. Add salt, ginger, onions, soy sauce, and water; cook for 2 minutes

7. Please the coconut rice in an eating bowl and top off with the ginger stir fry mix and hot sauce

- Calories: 400

- Fat: 16g

- Carbs: 42g

- Protein: 6g

Bok Choy Medley

Serves: 1

Preparation Time: 40 Minutes

Ingredients

- 1 Cup of Rice

- 1 Tablespoon of Apple Cider Vinegar

- 1/3 Cup of Honey

- ½ Teaspoon of Black Pepper

- ½ Teaspoon of Cayenne Powder

- 1 Diced Bok Choy

- 1 Cup of Fajita Peppers

- Onions to taste

Directions

1. Preheat oven to 350 degrees Fahrenheit

2. Pour rice into a dish and add vinegar and honey

3. Add bok choy, fajitas, onions, black pepper, and cayenne powder over the rice

4. Cover up with a foil and cook for a half hour

Nutritional Value

- Calories: 101

- Fat: 11g

- Carbs: 13mg

- Proteins: 5g

Avocado Tacos

Serves: 4

Preparation Time: 15 Minutes

Ingredients

- Corn Tortillas

- 1 Avocado

- 2 Tablespoons of Inions

- 1/8 Teaspoon of Garlic

- 1 Teaspoon of Lemon Juice

- Olive Oil to Taste

- 2 Tablespoons of Tomatoes
- 2 Teaspoons of Cilantro
- Salt and Pepper to taste
- ½ Clove of Garlic
- ¼ Cup of Black Beans

Directions

1. Preheat your oven to 325 degrees Fahrenheit
2. Heat olive oil over a medium flame
3. Add onions and garlic and cook for 3 minutes
4. Lower heat and add black beans
5. Set out tortillas on a baking sheet and heat in oven for 2 minutes
6. Mix avocado, garlic, lemon juice, salt and pepper, and olive oil in a bowl
7. Spread this mixture over the tortillas, and add onions and garlic, black beans, and cilantro before serving

Nutritional Value

- Calories: 377
- Fat: 18g
- Carbs: 44g

- Protein 9g

Mex Stackers

Serves: 8

Preparation Time: 25 Minutes

Ingredients

- 10 Tortilla Shells

- 2 Cups of Salsa

- 1/3 Cup of Turmeric Powder

- ½ Can of Black Beans

- 1 Package of Mexican Cheese

Directions

1. Preheat Oven to 350 Degrees Fahrenheit

2. Mix turmeric powder, black beans, and salsa in a bowl

3. Cut 3 inch circles out of the tortillas

4. Add a spoonful of the mixture over each tortilla circle and cover with cheese

5. Bake for 15 minutes and serve

Nutritional Value

- Calories: 234

- Fat: 25g

- Carbs: 43mg

- Protein: 3g

Quinoa Chard Pilaf

Serves: 3

Preparation Time: 25 Minutes

Ingredients

- 1 Teaspoon of Olive Oil

- 1 Tablespoon of Onion

- 1 Clove of Garlic

- ¼ Cup of Quinoa

- 2 Tablespoon of Lentils

- ½ Cup of Vegetable Broth

- ¼ Bunch of Swiss Chard

Directions

1. Heat oil in a pot over a medium flame

2. Add garlic and onion and stir together; sauté for 5 minutes

3. Add lentils and quinoa

4. Pour in broth

5. Cook for 15 minutes

6. Remove pot from the flame

7. Mix chard into the pot and cook for 5 more minutes before serving

Nutritional Value

- Calories: 150
- Fat: 3g

Nacho Muffins

Serves: 4

Preparation Time: 40 Minutes

Ingredients

- 1 Tablespoon of Olive Oil
- 1 Cup of Tomatoes
- 2 Scallions
- 1 Teaspoon of Basil
- 2 Teaspoons of Chili Powder
- 3 Ounces of Chicken
- 1 Cup of Mexican Cheese

Directions

1. Preheat oven to 350 Degrees Fahrenheit

2. Mix tortilla chips with olive oil in a processor

3. Press into molds on a muffin mold tray

4. Mix tomatoes, spices, scallions, and chicken in a bowl

5. Pour into the muffin molds

6. Bake for 30 minutes and serve

Nutritional Value

- Calories: 460

- Fat: 20g

- Carbs: 46mg

- Protein: 23g

Mediterranean Zucchini

Serves: 2

Preparation Time: 1 Hour

Ingredients

- 1 Teaspoon of Olive Oil

- 2 Tablespoon of Red Bell Pepper

- 2 Tablespoons of Onion

- 1 Clove of Garlic

- ¼ Cup of Tomatoes

- ¼ Cup of Cannellini Beans
- ½ Cup of Zucchini
- Salt and Pepper to Taste
- Water
- ¼ Cup of Rice

Directions

1. Pour water and rice into a pot over a high flame and cook until boiling

2. Reduce heat and allow it to simmer for 15 minutes

3. Heat olive oil in a saucepan over a medium heat

4. Add peppers, onions, and garlic, and cook for 5 minutes

5. Add zucchini, salt and pepper, oregano, and tomatoes and simmer for 20 minutes while stirring

6. Add beans and continue to cook for 10 minutes

7. Add in rice and serve

Nutritional Value

- Calories: 290
- Fat: 7.5g

Spring Rolls

Serves: 6

Preparation Time: 45 Minutes

Ingredients

- 6 Rice Paper Wrappers
- ½ Cup of Carrots
- ½ Cup of Cucumbers
- 1 Teaspoon of Vinegar
- 1 Cup of Avocado
- 1 Teaspoon of Lemon Juice
- ½ Tablespoon of Apple Cider Vinegar

Directions

1. Preheat Oven to 350 Degrees Fahrenheit

2. Lay out your wraps on the tray

3. Mix carrots, avocado, cucumber, lemon juice, vinegar, and apple cider vinegar together on a bowl

4. Add the mixture into each wrapper

5. Roll up the wrappers

6. Bake for 30 minutes and serve

Nutritional Value

- Calories: 123

- Fat: 3.2g

Hummus Zest

Serves: 2

Preparation Time: 15 Minutes

Ingredients

- 2/3 Cup of Chickpeas

- ½ Tablespoon of Olive Oil

- 1 Teaspoon of Red Peppers

- 1 Teaspoon of Oregano

- ½ Teaspoon of Thyme

Directions

1. Mix the oil, chickpeas, red pepper flakes, thyme, and oregano in a processor and process it

2. Store the mixture in a container in the refrigerator for up to three days or serve now

Nutritional Value

- Calories: 145
- Fat: 7.5g
- Protein: 8g

Mac and No Cheese

Serves: 4

Preparation Time: 1 Hour and 20 Minutes

Ingredients:

- ¾ Cup of Macaroni
- 1 Teaspoon of Olive Oil
- 1 Clove of Garlic
- ¼ Cup of Cashews
- 2 Tablespoons of Onion
- 2 Tablespoons of Red Peppers
- Water
- Salt and Pepper to Taste
- 1 Tablespoon of Lemon Juice
- ½ Teaspoon of Garlic Powder

- ½ teaspoon of Onion Powder

Directions

1. Preheat oven to 350 Degrees Fahrenheit

2. Boil a pot of salted water

3. Add pasta to the pot and cook for 10 minutes

4. Transfer to a baking dish

5. Heat olive oil in a saucepan and sauté onion and garlic for 4 minutes

6. Add macaroni and use a food processor to blend cashews, lemon juice, salt and pepper, and water together

7. 1 olive oil, garlic powder, onion powder, and red peppers together

8. Blend until mixed together

9. Combine the mixtures with the macaroni and bake for 45 minutes

10. Cool, add black peppers, and serve

Nutritional Value

- Calories: 207

- Fat: 10g

- Protein: 4g

Avocado Fries

Serves: 2

Preparation Time: 30 Minutes

Ingredients

• 3 Egg Whites

• 1/3 Cup of Bread Crumbs

• ½ Cup of Flower

• ¼ Cup of Parmesan

• 2 Avocados

Directions

1. Preheat oven to 425 Degrees Fahrenheit

2. Mix egg whites together and in a separate bowl mix breadcrumbs, cheese, and flower

3. Add avocado pieces into the egg mix and the flour mix separately

4. Place the avocado pieces on a baking tray

5. Bake for 20 minutes and serve

Nutritional Value

• Calories: 60

• Fat: 1.5g

• Carbs: 10mg

- Protein: 4.5g

Potato Curry

Serves: 3

Preparation Time: 40 Minutes

Ingredients

- 1 Teaspoon of Virgin Oil

- 2 Potatoes

- 1 Tablespoon of Onion

- 1 Clove of Garlic

- ½ Teaspoon of Ground Cumin

- ½ Teaspoon of Cayenne

- 2 Teaspoon of Ginger Root

- 1 Pinch of Salt

- 1 Tomato

- ¾ Teaspoon of Curry Powder

- ¼ Cup of Coconut Milk

Directions

1. Cut potato into cubes and place cubes in a pot with salt and water

2. Boil this over a high head, and then reduce heat and simmer for 15 minutes

3. Heat olive oil in a skillet and sauté garlic and onion for 5 minutes

4. Season with cumin, curry powder, cayenne pepper, ginger, and salt and pepper

5. Cook for 2 more minutes

6. Add beans, tomatoes, and more potatoes and pour in coconut milk

7. Simmer for 10 minutes and serve

Nutritional Value

- Calories: 280

- Fat: 16g

- Protein: 2g

- Carbs: 34g

Chicken-Celery Sticks

Serves: 1

Ingredients

- 4 Stalks of Celery

- 3 Ounces of Cream Cheese

- 2 Teaspoons of Basil

- 1/3 Cup of Chicken Cubes

Directions

1. Allow your cream cheese to sit for 30 minutes

2. Cut celery stocks into three pieces

3. Mix the stalks, basil, chicken cubes, and cream cheese in a bowl

4. Refrigerate for up to three days or serve now

Nutritional Value

- Calories: 35

- Fat: 6.5g

- Carbs: 3.5g

- Protein: 12.4g

Quinoa Chard Pilaf

Serves: 2

Preparation Time: 30 Minutes

Ingredients

- 1 teaspoon of olive oil

- 1 tablespoon of onions

- 1 clove of garlic

- ¼ cup of quinoa

- 2 tablespoon of lentils

- ½ cup of vegetable broth

- ¼ bunch of swiss chard

Directions

1. Heat the olive oil in a pot of a medium flame

2. Add onion and garlic and sauté for 5 minutes

3. Add lentils quinoa, and brother

4. Cook for 15 minutes

5. Get rid of head and shred chard into the pot

6. Cover pot and sit for 5 minutes

7. Serve

Nutritional Value

- Calories: 149

- Fat: 3g

Stuffed Peppers (No Meat)

Serves: 4

Preparation Time: 35 Minutes

Ingredients

- 1 Cup of Cauliflower

- ¾ Tablespoon of Melted Butter
- 1/3 Tablespoon of Garlic
- 4 Bell Peppers
- ½ Cup of Eggplant
- 1 Teaspoon of Basil
- ½ Teaspoon of Oregano

Directions

1. Preheat your oven to 350 Degrees Fahrenheit
2. Remove seeds from peppers and place in a dish
3. Process cauliflower, oil, butter, garlic, and puree in a food processor until mashed together
4. Place this mixture into peppers, and top with eggplant, oregano, basil, and cheese
5. Bake for 30 minutes and serve

Nutritional Value:

- Calories: 134

Veggie and Lentil Bake

Serves: 3

Preparation Time: 2 Hours

Ingredients

- ½ Cup of Rice
- Water
- 1 Cup of Lentils
- 1 Teaspoon of Olive Oil
- 1 Onion
- 3 Cloves of Garlic
- 1 Tomato
- 1/3 Cup of Celery
- 1 Teaspoon of Basil
- 1/3 Cup of Zucchini
- 1/3 Cup of Carrots
- 1 Can of Tomato
- 1 Teaspoon of Cumin
- ½ Teaspoon of Celery
- Salt and Pepper

Directions

1. Preheat your oven to 350 Degrees Fahrenheit

2. Mix oregano, basil, cumin, celery seeds, and salt and pepper in a bowl

3. Pour rice and water into a pot over a high flame and boil

4. Reduce heat and allow it to simmer for 20 minutes

5. Set lentils in a pot with more water and cook for 15 minutes over a medium to high heat

6. Heat oil in a skillet over a medium flame and add garlic and onion

7. Mix tomato, celery, carrots, tomato sauce, and zucchini together

8. Season with seasoning mix

9. In a dish, mix lentils, rice, and vegetables

10. Top off with tomato sauce, and sprinkle on more seasoning

11. Bake for 30 minutes in your oven

12. Remove and mix all of the mixtures together and serve

Nutritional Value

• Calories: 193

- Fat: 1.5g

- Carbs: 35g

- Protein: 10g

Grilled Tomato/Balsamic Veggie Dish

Serves: 4

Preparation Time: 30 Minutes

Ingredients

- 1 Teaspoon of Olive Oil

- ¼ Red Bell Pepper

- ¼ Zucchini

- ¼ Eggplant

- ¼ Sweet Onion

- 3 Tablespoons of Beans

- 2 Tomatoes

- 2 Teaspoons of Vinegar

- ¼ Cup of Couscous

- ¼ Cup of Vegetable Stock

Directions

1. Heat olive oil in a medium pan over a high flame

2. Add vegetables to the pan and turn sporadically; cook for 15 minutes

3. Add beans, tomatoes, and vinegar to vegetables and simmer for 5 minutes

4. Set couscous into a bowl and add vegetable stock

5. Stir for 3 minutes

6. Pour the couscous into a bowl and top off with the vegetable mixture

Nutritional Value

- Calories: 83
- Fat: 1.4g
- Carbs: 15g

Polenta Arepas (vegan)

Serves: 3

Preparation Time: 25 Minutes

Ingredients

- 8 Ounces of Tofu
- 16 Ounces of Polenta
- ½ Tablespoon of Olive Oil

- ½ Banana
- 1/4 Cup of Black Beans
- ½ Avocado
- 1 Tablespoon of Onion
- 1/4 Mango
- ¼ Jalapeno
- Salt and Pepper to taste

Directions

1. Preheat your oven's broiler
2. Slice up tofu and polenta and brush them with olive oil before arranging them and a baking sheet
3. Cook them in the broiler for 5 minutes
4. Heat olive oil in a skillet and sauté bananas for 5 minutes
5. Place black beans into a blender and process them until they have become a sauce
6. In a bowl, combine onion, mango, salt and pepper, and jalapeno
7. Set polenta and tofu on a plate and cover them with the bean sauce

8. Add bananas and the mixture; top off with salsa and serve

- Calories: 410
- Fat: 16g
- Carbs: 54g
- Protein: 14g

Chickpea Casserole

Serves: 3

Preparation Time: 1 Hour

Ingredients

- 1 Teaspoon of Olive Oil
- 1 Can of Chickpeas
- ½ Cup of Water
- ¼ Cup of White Wine
- 2 Teaspoons of Chili Powder
- 1 Teaspoon of Red Pepper Flakes
- 2 Cups of Rice

Directions

1. Drain out the beans and place all of the ingredients into a crock pot over a medium heat

2. Cook for 1 hour and serve

Nutritional Value

- Calories: 125

- Fat: 24g

- Carbs: 46mg

- Protein: 15g

Tempeh Fajitas

Serves: 2

Preparation Time: 15 Minutes

Ingredients

- 1 ½ Teaspoon of Olive Oil

- 8 Ounces of Olive Oil

- 2 Teaspoons of Soy Sauce

- 1 Teaspoon of Lime Juice

- 1 Tablespoon of Onion

- 1 Clove of Garlic

- 1/3 Cup of Green Bell Pepper

- ¾ Teaspoon of Green Peppers

- 1 Tablespoon of Cilantro
- 2 Tortillas

Directions

1. Preheat your oven to 350 Degrees Fahrenheit

2. Heat oil in a skillet over a medium flame

3. Add garlic and onion; sauté for 3 minutes

4. Add soy sauce, lime juice, and tempeh and cook until browned

5. Add chile peppers, bell peppers, and cilantro and cook for 10 minutes

6. Heat corn tortillas in oven for 3 minutes

7. Fill up the tortillas with the mixture and serve

Nutritional Value

- Calories: 155
- Fat: 4g

Chicken Teriyaki Stir Fry

Serves: 2

Preparation Time: Overnight

Ingredients

- 3 Ounces of Chicken Cubes

- 2 Teaspoons of Brown Sugar

- 1 Tablespoon of Honey

- 1 Cup of Rice

- 1/2 Cup of Bell Pepper Strips

- 1/3 Cup of Corn

Directions

1. Marinate the chicken cubes overnight in plastic bags in a marinade of brown sugar, sesame oil, and honey

2. Cook the next morning until complete and stir fry with corn, peppers, and rice; serve

Nutritional Value

- Calories: 97

- Fat: 14g

- Carbs: 32mg

- Protein 9g

Kale, Lentil, and Red Onion Pasta

Serves: 1

Preparation Time: 30 Minutes

Ingredients

- ½ Cup of Vegetable Broth

- 2 Tablespoons of Lentils

- Salt and Pepper to taste

- ½ Leaf of Bay

- 1 Tablespoon of Olive Oil

- ¼ Red Onion

- ¼ Teaspoon of Chopped Thyme

- 1 Teaspoon of Dried Oregano

- 1 Vegan Sausage

- ¼ Bunch of Kale

- 1 Cup of Rotini Pasta

Directions

1. Boil bay leaves, vegetable brother, salt and pepper, and lentils in a sauce pan over a high flame

2. Reduce heat and cook for twenty minutes

3. Add vegetable broth and discard the bay leaves

4. Heat olive oil in a separate skillet over a medium flame

5. Stir in thyme, onion, oregano, salt and pepper

6. Add sausage and reduce heat; cook for 10 minutes

7. Boil a pot of salted water and add rotini pasta and kale

8. Cook for 8 minutes

9. Drain the pasta and add in the onion mixture and lentils and serve

Nutritional Value

- Calories: 185
- Fat: 4g
- Carbs: 28g
- Protein: 9g

Butter Fettucine

Serves: 1

Preparation Time: 12 Minutes

Ingredients

• 4 Ounces of Fettucine

• ½ Tablespoon of Melted Butter

• 1 Teaspoon of Basil

• 1 Teaspoon of Thyme

• 1 Teaspoon of Oregano

Directions

1. Cook the fettucine for 8 minutes

2. Mix the melted butter with thyme, oregano, and basil

3. Pour this mixture over the fettucine and serve

Nutritional Value

• Calories: 104

• Fat: 8g

• Proteins: 8g

Teriyaki Tofu and Pineapple

Serves: 1

Preparation Time:

Ingredients

- 12 Ounces of Package Tofu

- 1/3 Cup of Pineapple

- ½ Cup of Teriyaki Sauce

- ¼ Cup of Rice

- Water

Directions

- Cut up the tofu and place in a dish

- Add pineapple and teriyaki sauce

- Cover and refrigerate for one hour

- Preheat oven to 350 degrees Fahrenheit

- Bake tofu for 20 minutes

- Place rice and water in a pot and boil over a high flame before reducing heating and simmering for 15 minutes

- Pour rice into a bowl and top off with the pineapple teriyaki tofu and serve

- Calories: 212
- Fat: 2g
- Protein: 6g
- Carbs: 43g

Tortillas and Rice

Serves: 2

Preparation Time: 1 Hour

Ingredients

- 2 Cups of Cooked Rice
- Olive Oil to taste
- ½ Tablespoon of Chili Powder
- ½ Teaspoons of Cumin
- 2 Tortilla Shells

Directions

1. Preheat oven to 400 degrees Fahrenheit

2. Place rice on a stove and add water and spices

3. Boil and then reduce the heat and simmer for 25 minutes while stirring

4. Set the tortilla shells over one another and cut into triangles

5. Set the tortilla pieces on the baking tray and cook for 22 minutes

6. Remove from tray, cover with the rest of the mixes, and serve

Nutritional Value:

• Calories: 84

• Carbs: 11mg

Tofu and Red Bell Peppers

Serves: 4

Preparation Time: 25 minutes

Ingredients

• 14 Ounces of Tofu

• ½ Tablespoon of Olive Oil

• ½ Tablespoon of Soy Sauce

• ½ Red Bell Pepper

• 1 Tablespoon of Onion

- ¾ Tablespoon of Peanut Butter

- ½ Tablespoon of Lime Juice

- 2 Teaspoons of Sriracha

- 2 Teaspoons of Brown Sugar

- Water

- ½ Tablespoons of Cilantro

Directions

1. Start by preheating your oven to 450 degrees Fahrenheit

2. Slice the tofu into four square like pieces

3. Whisk olive oil and soy sauce in a bowl

4. Coat the tofu in the resulting mixture

5. Place the pieces of tofu on a baking sheet and place onions and peppers alongside them

6. Bake for 10-15 minutes

7. In a pan over a low flame, mix together lime juice, peanut butter, chili sauce, brown sugar, soy sauce, and water; cook until warm

8. Remove the tofu, onions, and peppers from the oven and set in a bowl

9. Cover it with the new peanut butter mixture and top with cilantro if desired before serving

Nutritional Value

- Calories: 275
- Fat: 11g
- Carbs: 26.4g
- Protein 17.6g

Broccoli Curry

Serves: 2

Preparation Time: 40 Minutes

Ingredients

- ½ Tablespoon of Vegetable Oil
- 2/3 Cup of Broccoli
- 1 Cup of Rice
- ½ Cup of Water
- 1 Tablespoon of Coconut Milk
- 2 Tablespoons of Turmeric

Directions

1. Pour oil in a pot over a medium flame and sauté broccoli and tofu for 3 minutes

2. Add water, rice, coconut milk, and boil

3. Lower heat and simmer for 30 minutes

4. Stir in rice and serve

Nutritional Value

- Calories: 90

- Protein: 24g

Risotto

Serves: 2

Preparation Time: 20 Minutes

Ingredients

- 3 Ounces of Ham (low sodium)

- 1 Tablespoon of Butter

- 1 Tablespoon of Olive Oil

- 2 Cups of Rice

- 1 Cup of Vegetable Bouillon

- 1/3 Teaspoon of Black Pepper

- ¼ Teaspoon of Orange Peel

- 2 Scallions

Directions

1. Melt butter and pour it into olive oil in a skillet over a medium heat

2. Pour in uncooked rice and stir it for 5 minutes

3. Add the ham, spices, and bullion

4. Increase the heat and bring the mixture to a boil

5. Top off with scallions and serve

Nutritional Value

- Calories: 312
- Fat: 24g

Almond and Quinoa Salad

Serves: 1

Preparation Time: 30 Minutes

Ingredients

- 3 Tablespoons of Almonds
- ¼ Cup of Quinoa
- Water

- 2 Teaspoons of Olive Oil

- ½ Yellow Bell Pepper

- 1 Clove of Garlic

- Salt and Pepper

- Lime Juice

Directions

1. Preheat oven to 350 Degrees Fahrenheit

2. Set the almonds on a baking sheet and bake in the oven for seen minutes

3. In a pan over a medium flame, heat a teaspoon of olive oil

4. Add garlic, scallions, yellow pepper, and red pepper flakes and cook for five minutes

5. Add salt and pepper, water, thyme, and quinoa and boil before reducing heat of flame to simmer for 7 minutes

6. Add in zucchini and stir and cook for five more minutes

7. Remove the pan from the heat and add celery, almonds, and olive oil

8. Season with salt and pepper and continue to stir before serving

Nutritional Information

- Calories: 278
- Fat: 8g
- Protein: 8g

Tofu Fajitas

Serves: 4

Preparation Time: 15 Minutes

Ingredients

- 4 Tortilla Shells
- ½ Tablespoon of Butter
- 1 Tablespoon of Coconut Oil
- 1 Onion
- 2 Bell Peppers
- 1 Block of Tofu
- 2 Teaspoons of Lemon Juice
- 1 Teaspoon of Cayenne Pepper
- ½ Teaspoon of Cumin

Directions

1. Warm the shells in a skillet for 2 minutes

2. Cut the onions, tofu, and peppers into strips

3. Slather them with butter in a large pot and cook over a high heat for 3 minutes

4. Add this mixture over the shells and serve

Nutritional Value

- Calories: 210
- Fat: 17g

Vegan Chili

Serves: 3

Preparation Time: 30 Minutes

Ingredients

- 2 Tablespoons of Olive Oil
- 1 Onion
- 4 Cloves of Garlic
- 1 ½ Teaspoon of Cumin
- 1 Teaspoon of Chili Powder
- Salt and Pepper
- 1 Zucchini

- ¾ Cup of Tomato Paste
- 15 Ounces of Black Beans
- 15 Ounces of Pinto Beans
- 1 can of Tomatoes
- Water

Directions

1. Heat the olive oil in a pot over a high flame
2. Add garlic and onion and cook for 4 minutes
3. Add chili powder, cumin, and salt and pepper
4. Add zucchini and tomato paste and cook for 3 minutes
5. Add black and pinto beans and tomatoes, and two cups of water
6. Boil the resulting mixture
7. Bring heat down and simmer the mixture for 20 minutes
8. Serve

Nutritional Information

- Calories: 236
- Fat: 4g

Veggie Burger with Cucumber Salad

Serves: 1

Preparation Time: 20 Minutes

Ingredients

- 1 Ciabatta Roll
- 1 Veggie Burger
- 1 Teaspoon of Brown Sugar
- 1 Teaspoon of Thyme
- 1 Onion
- 1 Cucumber
- 4 Cherry Tomatoes
- 3 Cups of Olive Oil
- 1 Shallot
- 1 Tablespoon of White Wine Vinegar
- ½ Tablespoon of Basil

Directions

1. Cut the cucumbers into crescent shapes and then cut the cherry tomatoes in half

2. Slice the onions into strips

3. Place the onion strips, cucumbers, and cherry tomatoes into a bowl and mix it with basic, vinegar, and olive oil to form a salad

4. Cover up the salad and store it in a refrigerator

5. Mix brown sugar and thyme and sprinkle it over a veggie burger

6. Cook the burger until complete

7. Retrieve the salad from the refrigerator and serve it alongside the veggie burger

Nutritional Value

• Calories: 217

Sesame Tofu and Broccoli

Serves: 1

Preparation Time: 20 Minutes

Ingredients

• ½ Block of Tofu

• 1 Tablespoon of Sesame Seeds

• ¼ Tablespoon of Sesame Oil

- ¾ Tablespoon of Soy Sauce

- 1 Cup of Broccoli

- Salt and Pepper

- Water

Directions

- Slice the tofu into two pieces and then into two pieces each to make four pieces total

- Spread out all of your sesame seeds out on a plate

- Press all sides of the tofu pieces into the square

- Heat sesame oil in a skillet over a medium flame

- Cook the tofu for five minutes on each side in the skillet

- Add in soy sauce and cook for one more minute

- Remove the tofu from the skillet, and then add water, broccoli, and salt and paper into the skillet and cook for five minutes

• Place the tofu and broccoli on an eating plate and serve

Nutritional Value

• Calories: 148

• Fat: 5g

• Carbs: 18g

• Protein: 14g

Pot Pie Muffin

Serves: 1

Preparation Time: 25 Minutes

Ingredients

• 3 Ounces of White Chicken Meat

• 1 Cup of Cauliflower

• ½ Cup of Chicken Bouillon

• 1/3 Cup of Vegetable Mix

• 1 Teaspoon of Garlic

• 1/8 Teaspoon of Sage

Directions

• Preheat oven to 375 degrees Fahrenheit

- Place cauliflower in a food processor and process
- In a bowl mix together mash, seasonings, and chicken
- Set the dough on a flat surface and cut it up into holes that can fit in a muffin mold tray
- Fill up each muffin with a spoonful of the mixture
- Bake for 20 minutes and serve

Nutritional Value

- Calories: 321

Stuffed Sweet Potatoes

Serves: 1

Preparation Time: 1 Hour

Ingredients

- 1 Sweet Potato
- ¼ Tablespoon of Olive Oil
- ¼ Onion
- 1 Clove of Garlic

- ½ Teaspoon of Rosemary
- 1 Pinch of Red Pepper Flakes
- Salt and Pepper to Taste
- 1 Cup of Kale
- 2 Ounces of Tofu
- Water

Directions

- Preheat your oven to 375 degrees Fahrenheit
- Bake your sweet potato on a baking sheet for 1 hour, but keep the oven on
- Cut off the top quarter of the potato and throw it away to leave a shell
- Heat oil in a skillet over a high flame and add onion, rosemary, salt and pepper, garlic, and red pepper flakes
- Cook while stirring for 3 minutes
- Add kale and cook for 5 more minutes
- Add in sweet potato, tofu, and water
- Cook for 1 more minute
- Place the entire meal on baking sheet and bake it for 30 minutes before serving

- Calories: 190
- Fat: 4.5g

Veggie Pita

Serves: 1

Preparation Time: 15 Minutes

Ingredients

- 1 Pita Pocket
- 1 Teaspoon of Paprika
- ¼ Teaspoon of Black Pepper
- 1/3 Cup of Bok Choy Pieces
- 1/3 Cup of Avocado Pieces
- 1/3 Cup of Cucumber
- 1/3 Cup of Carrots
- 1/3 Cup of Tomatoes
- 1 Teaspoon of Lemon Juice

Directions

1. Begin heating your boiler

2. Place the vegetables into a bowl and add lemon juice and spices

3. Mix the vegetables and spices together well

4. Spoon this mix inside the pita and cook in the broiler for 5 minutes before serving

Nutritional Value

- Calories: 312

- Fat: 23mg

- Carbs: 68mg

Tofu Kebabs and Cilantro

Serves: 2

Preparation Time: 25 Minuets

Ingredients

- ½ Cup of Cilantro

- 1 Tablespoon of Olive Oil

- ¼ Jalapeno

- 1 Teaspoon of Ginger

- ½ Tablespoon of Lime Juice

- 1 Scallion

- Salt and Pepper
- 7 Ounces of Tofu
- ½ Squash

Directions:

1. Heat up your grill to medium heat

2. Combine oil, cilantro, jalapeno, ginger, juice, and scallion together in a processor

3. Blend until the mixture is smooth and then add salt and pepper

4. In a bowl, combine tofu, scallions, and olive oil

5. Place the scallions and tofu into a skewer and then the squash into another skewer

6. Grill the resulting squash kebab for 12 minutes over the grill and the tofu kebab for 7 minutes

7. Season with cilantro and serve

Nutritional Value

- Calories: 255
- Fat: 10g
- Carbs: 27g

Chicken Nuggets and Chinese Veggie Salad

Serves: 1

Preparation Time: 30 minutes

Ingredients

- 3 Ounces of Chicken Meat
- 2 Egg Whites
- Salt and Pepper
- 2 Cups of Cabbage
- Salt and Pepper
- 1 Stalk of Bok Choy
- 3 Ounces of bean Sprouts

Directions

1. Preheat Oven to 375 Degrees Fahrenheit

2. Scramble up your eggs in a bowl, and then your seasoning and breadcrumbs in another mixture

3. Run the chicken through the egg coating and the breadcrumb/seasoning coating

4. Set the chicken on a baking tray and cook for 25 minutes and then serve

Nutritional Value

- Calories: 560

Vegan Salad

Serves: 2

Preparation Time: 2 Hours

Ingredients:

- ¼ Cup of Amaranth

- 1/2 Cup of Vegetable Broth

- ½ Cup of Quinoa

- ¼ Teaspoon of Orange Zest

- ¼ Cup of Orange Segments

- ¼ Cup of Fennel

- ¼ Cup of Radishes

- 1 Tablespoon of Olive Oil

- 2 Tablespoon of Orange Juice

- ½ Tablespoon of Red Wine Vinegar

- Salt and Pepper

Directions

1. Cook the amaranth by placing it in a pan over a high flame and toasting for five minutes

2. In a separate pan, bring a half cup of vegetable broth to a broil

3. Transfer the amaranth to the vegetable broth pain and simmer for seven minutes after reducing the flame

4. Remove pan from heat

5. Cook quinoa by also placing it in a pan of boiled vegetable broth and add salt and pepper; simmer for 10 minutes under a reduced heat after boiling

6. Cook the millet by placing it in yet another pan over a medium to high flame and cooking for five minutes

7. Pour the millet into a bowl and mix it with cold water

8. Bring more vegetable brother to a boil in another pan

9. Add the millet and salt to the brother and simmer for 15 minutes

10. Merge all of the ingredients into one bowl and refrigerate for 1 hour before serving

Nutritional Value

- Calories: 380
- Fat: 7g
- Carbs: 68g
- Protein: 11g

Pizza (Gout Friendly Version)

Serves: 2

Preparation Time: 30 Minutes

Ingredients

- 2 Tablespoons of Olive Oil
- 1 Cup of Feta Cheese
- 4 Cups of Cherry Tomatoes
- 1 Cup of Radish
- 1 Cup of Avocado
- 1 Teaspoon of Red Pepper Flakes
- 1 Tablespoon of Basil Leaves
- 1 Teaspoon of Oregano

- Pizza Dough (enough as needed)

Directions

- Flatten out the pizza dough and cover it with olive oil, seasoning and cheese
- Add the rest of the ingredients and bake according to the instructions on the dough package

Nutritional Value

- Calories: 225
- Fat: 7g

Barley and Winter Green Pesto

Serves: 2

Preparation Time: 45 Minutes

Ingredients

- ½ Cup of Barley
- Water
- ½ Bunch of Swiss Chard
- ½ Bunch of Mustard Greens
- 2 Tablespoons of Almonds

- 1 ½ Teaspoon of Vinegar
- 1 Clove of Garlic
- 1 ½ Tablespoon of Walnut Oil
- Salt and Pepper

Directions

- Set the barley and salt and pepper on a pan
- Boil the pan over a high heat, and then reduce the heat and simmer for 30 minutes
- Drain the pan and then fill up another pan with salted water and boil it as well
- Add chard and mustard green to this pan and simmer for 1 minute
- Drain the second pan
- Mix greens, vinegar, almonds, and garlic in a food processor and process
- Add walnut oil into the mix and continue to process for 2 more minutes
- Mix all of the ingredients together and add pesto and barley and more salt and pepper as desired before serving

- Calories: 315
- Fat: 14g
- Carbs: 37g

Garbanzo Cake and Avocado

Serves: 4

Preparation Time: 35 Minutes

Ingredients

- ¼ Cup of Bulgur Wheat
- Water
- ¼ Cup of Parsley Leaves
- 14 Cup of Mint Leaves
- ¼ Cup of Cilantro Leaves
- 1 Clove of Garlic
- 1/4 Teaspoon of Coriander
- ½ Jalapeno Chili
- ½ Can of Garbanzo beans
- ¼ Cup of Olive Oil
- ¼ Avocado

- ½ Tablespoon of Lime Juice

- Breadcrumbs

Directions

- Bring a cup of water to a boil

- Ad bulgur wheat and cook for 10 minutes, and then drain

- Mix parsley, cilantro, mint, garlic, jalapeno peppers, and coriander together in a food processor and process

- Add half of the garbanzo beans and pulse again

- Transfer the bean mixture to a bowl and add chickpeas and process again.

- Transfer to the same bowl

- Add bulgur wheat to the bowl as well

- Season the chickpea/bean/wheat mixture in the bowl with salt and pepper

- Fold the mixture with a spatula

- Cut the mix into patties with each patty being an inch wide

- Combine flour and water together in a second bowl and mix it together until smooth
- Dip each patty in the mixture to coat it thoroughly and then cover both sides with breadcrumbs
- Transfer the patties to a plate and cook in a skillet over a medium flame for about 2-3 minutes on each side
- Season again with salt and pepper and limejuice, and serve alongside mashed avocado and onions

Nutritional Information

- Calories: 700
- Fat: 28g
- Carbohydrates: 96g
- Protein: 15g

Veggie Burger Quesadilla

Serves: 1

Preparation Time: 10 Minutes

Ingredients

- 2 burrito tortillas
- 3 ounces of veggie burger
- ¼ Cup of Mexican cheese
- ½ cup of scallions
- 1 teaspoons of chili
- ½ teaspoon of cumin
- 1 teaspoon of cilantro
- 1 tablespoon of Mexican seasoning

Directions

1. Set a skillet over a medium to high flame

2. Layer the ingredients between the two tortillas to make a quesadilla

3. Cook the quesadilla on both sides in the skillet, with at least four minutes per side

4. Remove and serve

Nutritional Value

- Calories: 134

Vegan Paella

Serves: 1

Preparation Time: 40 Minutes

Ingredients:

* Water

* ¼ Cup of Rice

* ¾ Teaspoons of Olive Oil

* ¼ Onion

* 1 Clove of Garlic

* ¼ Green Bell Pepper

* ¼ Red Bell Pepper

* ½ Tomato

* ¼ Cup of Vegetable Broth

* 1 Teaspoon of Paprika

* ½ Teaspoon of Turmeric

* ¼ Cup of Beas

* ¼ Cup of Artichoke Hearts

* Salt and Pepper

Directions

1. Mix the water and rice together in a bowl and let it sit for 20 minutes before draining

2. Heat the olive oil in a skillet over a medium flame and stir it for five minutes with onion and garlic

3. Add red bell and green bell peppers and tomato

4. Cook and stir for 3 minutes

5. Add rice and vegetable brother into the mixture and boil

6. Reduce heat and allow to simmer, with an addition of paprika and turmeric, for 20 more minutes

7. Add salt and pepper, peas, and artichoke hearts into the rice mixture and stir for 1 minute

8. Merge all remaining ingredients and serve

Nutritional Value

- Calories: 125
- Carbs: 26g

Celery Root Soup

Serves: 2

Preparation Time: 20 Minutes

Ingredients

- 3 Tablespoons of Olive Oil

- 1 Cup of Celery Root

- 2 Potatoes

- 1 Apple

- 2 Cloves of Garlic

- Salt and Pepper

- Water

- 2 Cups of Vegetable Broth

Directions

1. Heat the olive oil in a pan with a lid over a medium flame

2. Add celery roots, potatoes, garlic, salt and pepper, and apple and cook for three minutes

3. Add water and broth and increase temperature to a boil

4. Reduce heat and simmer the vegetables for twenty minutes

5. Pour the soup into a blender and puree it

6. Once the soup has been blended, transfer it back to the pan and warm it over a low heat

7. Add more salt and pepper, and serve

Nutritional Value

- Calories: 150
- Fat: 4g
- Carbs: 27g

Spicy Quinoa and Edamame

Serves: 1

Preparation Time:

Ingredients

- Water
- ½ Cup of Quinoa
- 1 Teaspoon of Vegetable Bouillon
- ¾ Cup of Edamame
- 1 Teaspoon of Olive Oil
- ½ Sweet Onion
- ½ Bell Pepper

- 1 ½ Teaspoon of Ginger
- 2 Cloves of garlic
- 1 Tablespoon of Soy Sauce
- 2 Teaspoon of Cilantro
- 1 Teaspoon of Hot Sauce

Directions

1. Mix vegetable bouillon, quinoa, and water together in a pot over a medium flame

2. Add in edamame and simmer for 15 minutes

3. Heat up olive oil over a medium flame and add in peppers and onions and cook for 5 minutes

4. Add in garlic and ginger and cook for 2 minutes

5. Add in soy sauce, chili paste, and cilantro and continue to mix for 5 more minutes

6. Merge all ingredients and serve

Nutritional Value

- Calories: 166

Roast Beef Wraps

Serves: 1

Preparation Time: 5 Minutes

Ingredients

- 1 Sandwich Wrap

- 3 Ounces of Roast Beef

- 1 Tablespoon of Onion Dip Powder

- 1 Roasted Pepper

- 1 Tomato

- 1 Tablespoon of Apple Cider Vinegar

- 1 Teaspoon of Lemon Juice

- 1 Red Pepper

Directions

1. Layout your sandwich wrap

2. Mix the onion dip powder, mushrooms, veggie slices, apple cider vinegar, lemon juice, and red pepper flakes in a bowl

3. Lay your roast beef on the wrap and then place the above mixture on top

4. Roll up the wrap and enjoy

- Calories: 112
- Fat: 0.4mg

Black Eyed Peas and Collard Greens and Turnips

Serves:

Preparation Time: Overnight

Ingredients

- ¼ Cup of Rice
- Water
- ½ Cup of Peas
- 1 Teaspoon of Margarine (soy)
- ½ Turnip
- 1 Tomato
- 1 Teaspoon of Balsamic Vinaigrette Salad Dressing
- ¼ Bunch of Greens

Directions

1. Place the peas into a container and cover it with water and allow it to sit overnight

2. In the morning, prepare your rice by placing the rice and a small cup of water into a small pot

3. Boil the rice over a high flame, and then simmer it for 15 minutes

4. Cover up the peas that were soaked in water overnight with new water

5. Boil it over a high heat, and then simmer it over a medium flame for 40 minutes

6. Heat the soy margarine in a skillet and add greens and turnip and salt and pepper cook for 3 minutes

7. Combine the two mixtures and stir for 5 minutes

Nutritional Value

- Calories; 160
- Carbs: 31g

Honeyed Corn

Serves: 4

Preparation Time: 30 Minutes

Ingredients

• 4 Ears of Corn

• 3 Tablespoons of Honey

• 1 Tablespoon of Melted Butter

• 2/3 Tablespoon of Apple Cider Vinegar

• 1 Tablespoon of Turmeric

Directions

1. Mix the honey, vinegar, melted butter, and turmeric in a bowl

2. Coat each corn ear with the mixture

3. Wrap the corn ears and grill for twenty minutes over a medium heat

4. Serve

Nutritional Value

• Calories: 38

• Fat: 17g

• Carbs: 43g

• Protein: 6g

Black Bean Quesadilla (Vegan Version)

Serves: 1

Preparation Time: 30 Minutes

Ingredients

- ¼ Cup of Black Beans
- 4 Tablespoons of Tomatoes
- 1 Clove of Garlic
- ½ Teaspoon of Cumin
- 1 Pinch of Chili Powder
- 1 Pinch of Cayenne Pepper
- Salt and Pepper
- 2 Tortillas
- 1 Tablespoon of Cilantro
- 1 Teaspoon of Olive Oil

Directions

1. Blend the beans, tomatoes, and garlic in a processor and blend until smooth

2. Add chili powder, cayenne pepper, salt and pepper, and cumin and blend until smooth again

3. Transfer this mixture to a bowl and add a tablespoon of tomatoes and cilantro

4. Heat the olive oil in a skillet and then set the first tortilla over the oil

5. Spread your mixture over the tortilla, and then place another tortilla over it

6. Cook the tortilla for 5-10 minutes and flip at least twice

7. Serve

Nutritional Value

• Calories: 122

Baked Tofu and Roasted Pepper

Serves: 1

Preparation Time: 25 Minutes

Ingredients

• ½ Diced Shallot

• ¼ Container of Tofu

• Water

• 1 Tablespoon of White Wine

• 1 Teaspoon of Red Pepper Slices

Directions

1. Preheat your oven to four hundred degrees Fahrenheit

2. Pour the water, peppers, tofu, and shallots into a pot and bake for twenty minutes before serving

Nutritional Value

• Calories: 56

• Carbs: 14mg

• Protein: 8g

Red Bell Pepper (stuffed)

Serves: 1

Preparation Time: 45 Minutes

Ingredients

• ¼ Cup of Brown Rice

• Water

• 1 Red Bell Pepper

• ¼ Onion

- 1 Clove of Garlic
- 4 Ounces of Black Eyed Peas
- 1 Leaf of Swiss Chard
- Salt and Pepper

Directions

- Preheat your oven to 350 degrees Fahrenheit
- Boil brown rice and water in a pan over a high heat
- Reduce the heat and simmer for 15 minutes
- Set red pepper on a baking sheet and bake for 15 minutes
- Heat olive oil in a skillet and then add garlic and onion, and stir for 5 minutes
- Add the peas and chard, and cook for 5 more minutes
- Mix in the brown rice, season with salt and pepper, and stuff this mix into the red pepper
- Serve

Nutritional Value

- Calories: 100
- Carbs: 21

Baked Pepper Taquitos

Serves: 6

Preparation Time: 1 Hour

Ingredients

• 6 Tortillas

• 1/3 Cup of Monterey Jack Cheese

• 1 Cup of Tomatoes

• 1 Jalapeno Pepper

• 1 Teaspoon of Chili Powder

• 1/3 Teaspoon of Cumin

• ½ Teaspoon of Celery Flakes

• Olive Oil to Taste

• Your Choice of Chicken or Pork

Directions

• Either use leftover chicken or pork or cook new meat now

• Shred apart your choice of meat and preheat your oven to 350 Degrees Fahrenheit

• Lay tortillas on a baking tray and mix together the protein, cheese, tomatoes, peppers, and spices

- Pour this mixture over your tortillas and then add the meat

- Roll and bake for 30 Minutes

- Serve

Nutritional Value

- Calories: 105

White Beans and Chard

Serves: 2

Preparation Time: 20 Minutes

Ingredients

- ¼ Bunch of Swiss Chard

- 1 Tablespoon of Olive Oil

- ¼ Onion

- 1 Clove of Garlic

- Salt and pepper to taste

- 7 ounces of cannellini beans

- ½ Cup of Vegetable Broth

- 1 Tablespoon of parsley

- 1 teaspoon of white wine vinegar

Directions

1. Remove the stems from the chard leaves

2. Stack up the leaves and cut them into small pieces

3. Heat the olive oil in a pan over a medium flame until it shimmers

4. Add the chard stems, garlic, onion, and salt and pepper to taste

5. Cook and stir for 8 minutes

6. Then, add the chard leaves, beans, salt, and broth and stir for 5 more minutes

7. Remove from the oven and add in vinegar and parsley to taste before serving

Nutritional Value

- Calories: 185
- Fat: 9g
- Carbs: 21g

Baked Chicken Wings

Serves: 1

Preparation Time: 3 Hours

Ingredients

• 3 Ounces of Chicken Wings

• 1 Cup of Molasses

• ½ Cup of Ketchup

• 1 Tablespoon of Mustard

• ½ Tablespoon of Honey

• 2/3 Tablespoon of Hot Sauce

• 3 Teaspoons of Cayenne Powder

• 1 Jalapeno Pepper

Directions

1. Combine ketchup, molasses, honey, mustard, hot sauce, and spices together and boil over a high flame before reducing the flame and simmering for half an hour to create a sauce

2. Prepare your crock pot and then insert the chicken

3. Pour the sauce over the chicken

4. Bake for two hours before serving

Nutritional Value

- Calories: 105

Miso Soup and Napa Cabbage

Serves: 1

Preparation Time: 30 Minutes

Ingredients

- 1 Teaspoon of Olive Oil

- ¼ Onion

- 1 Teaspoon of Ginger

- 1 Clove of Garlic

- 1/ ½ Cups of Vegetable Broth

- ½ Tablespoon of Soy Sauce

- 6 Ounces of Noodles

- ¼ Cabbage

- ½ Carrot

- ¼ Cup of Hot Sauce

Directions

1. Bring a pot of salted water to boiling over a high flame

2. Add noodles to the water and cook according to the directions listed on the package

3. Drain out of the water

4. Heat the oil in a pan over a medium heat until it is shimmering, and then add ginger, garlic, carrot, and onion and cook for 5 minutes

5. Increase the heat and add soy sauce and broth and stir thoroughly

6. Add cabbage and stir and cook for 5 minutes

7. Add all of the ingredients together and season with salt and pepper as desired before serving

Nutritional Value

- Calories: 131
- Carbs: 24g

Stuffed Pepper Melt

Serves: 1

Preparation Time: 30 Minutes

Ingredients

- 4 Bell Peppers

- 1 Tablespoon of Coconut Oil

- 1 Cup of Cauliflower

- Scallions

- 1 Tablespoon of Mushrooms

- 1 Jalapeno Pepper

- 1 Cup of Monterey Jack Cheese

Directions

1. Preheat oven to 325 degrees Fahrenheit

2. Mix together all of the ingredients except for the cheese in a bowl

3. Spoon this mixture into the peppers

4. Top off with cheese and bake for 25 minutes before serving

Nutritional Value

- Calories: 108

- Fat: 13mg

- Carbs: 36mg

- Protein: 12g

Chinese Porridge (Vegan Version)

Serves: 3

Preparation Time: One Hour and a Half

Ingredients

• Water

• ½ Cup of Vegetable Broth

• ½ Cup of Rice

• ¼ Piece of Ginger

• Salt and Pepper

• 1 Cup of Kale

Directions

1. Place all of the ingredients except for the kale into a pan and boil it over a high flame

2. Reduce the flame and then simmer while stirring for one and a half hours

3. Shut off the heat and add the kale

4. Stir and cook for 5 minutes

5. Add more salt and pepper as desired and serve

Nutritional Value

• Calories: 146

• Carbs: 31g

Roasted Chicken and White Pepper

Serves: 5

Preparation Time: One Hour and 30 Minutes

Ingredients

• 5 Pounds or Chicken

• 1/3 Cup of Olive Oil

• ½ Tablespoon of Sage

• 1 Teaspoon of White Pepper

• 1 Teaspoon of Rosemary

• 1 Teaspoon of Orange

Directions

1. Preheat oven to 350 degrees Fahrenheit

2. Place chicken in a dish

3. Mix oil, sage, oranges, peppers, and rosemary in a bowl and cook for one and a half hours before serving

Nutritional Value

• Calories: 207

- Fat: 33mg

- Carbs: 56mg

Swiss Chard and Garbanzo Beans

Serves: 3

Preparation Time: 30 Minutes

Ingredients:

- 2 Tablespoons of Nuts

- 4 Tablespoons of Couscous

- 1 Tablespoon of Olive Oil

- 1 Clove of Garlic

- 5 Tablespoons of Garbanzo Beans

- 2 Tablespoons of Raisins

- ¼ Bunch of Swiss Chard

- Salt and Pepper

Directions

1. Set the couscous in a bowl and add water

2. Stir for 10 minutes

3. Cover this mixture and cook over a medium flame

4. While it is cooking, toast your nuts in a skillet over a low heat for 3 minutes

5. Heat olive oil in a skillet and add garlic, garbanzo beans, raisings, salt and pepper, and chard

6. Cook for 5 minutes

7. Fluff the couscous and place in a bowl; then top with previous mixture and nuts

Nutritional Value

- Calories: 142
- Fat: 6g
- Carbs: 18g

Garbanzo Curry

Serves: 3

Preparation Time: 45 Minutes

Ingredients:

- ¾ Teaspoon of Olive Oil
- ¼ Onion
- ½ Clove of Garlic

- ¼ Teaspoon of Ginger Root
- 1/8 Teaspoon of Cinnamon
- 1/8 Teaspoon of Cumin
- 1.8 Teaspoon of Coriander
- 1/8 Teaspoon of Cayenne Pepper
- ¼ Can of Garbanzo Beans
- 1/8 Teaspoon of Ground Turmeric
- 2 Tablespoons of Cilantro
- ¼ Cup of Rice
- Water

Directions

1. Place water and rice in a pot and boil over a high heat

2. Reduce heat and simmer for 15 minutes

3. Heat olive oil in a skillet over a medium heat

4. Saute onions in olive oil for 3 minutes

5. Add garlic, ginger, cinnamon, cumin, salt and pepper, cayenne, coriander, and turmeric and cook for 1 minute while stirring

6. Add beans and water and cook for 15 minutes

7. Place rice in a bowl and top off with the mixture and cilantro

Nutritional Value

- Calories: 295
- Fat: 4.5g
- Carbs: 57g
- Protein: 7g

Peaches with Berry Sauce Ice Cream

Serves: 1

Preparation Time: 5 Minutes

Ingredients

- Berry Sauce of your choice
- Sliced Peaches
- 1 Tablespoon of Honey
- 1 Teaspoon of Lemon Juice
- Low Fat Ice Cream of Your Choice

Directions

1. Scoop up ice cream in a bowl

2. Top off with all of the other ingredients and serve

- Calories: 150

www.ingramcontent.com/pod-product-compliance
Lightning Source LLC
Chambersburg PA
CBHW071218240726
48654CB00009B/832